Taking Care of Myself

Hygiene

By Meg Gaertner

level 2
little blue readers

www.littlebluehousebooks.com

Little Blue House is distributed by North Star Editions:
sales@northstareditions.com | 888-417-0195

Produced for Little Blue House by Red Line Editorial.

Photographs ©: Shutterstock Images, cover, 4, 6, 9, 10–11, 13, 14, 16–17, 19 (top), 19 (bottom), 20–21, 23, 24 (top left), 24 (top right), 24 (bottom left), 24 (bottom right)

Library of Congress Control Number: 2021916794

ISBN
978-1-64619-493-3 (hardcover)
978-1-64619-520-6 (paperback)
978-1-64619-571-8 (ebook pdf)
978-1-64619-547-3 (hosted ebook)

Printed in the United States of America
Mankato, MN
012022

About the Author

Meg Gaertner enjoys reading, writing, dancing, and being outside. She lives in Minnesota.

Table of Contents

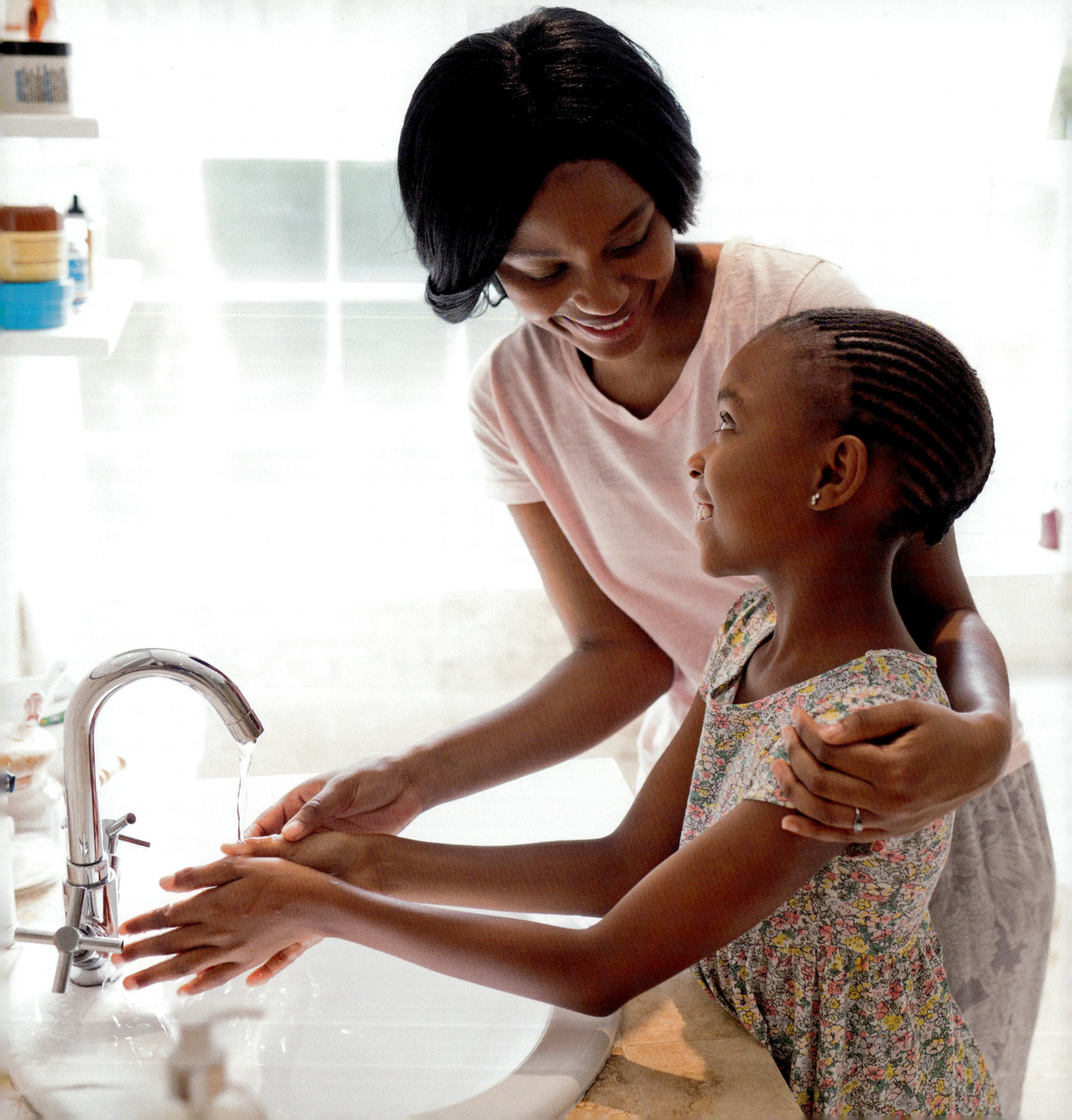

Hygiene

Actions to stay clean are called hygiene.
Good hygiene helps people stay healthy.

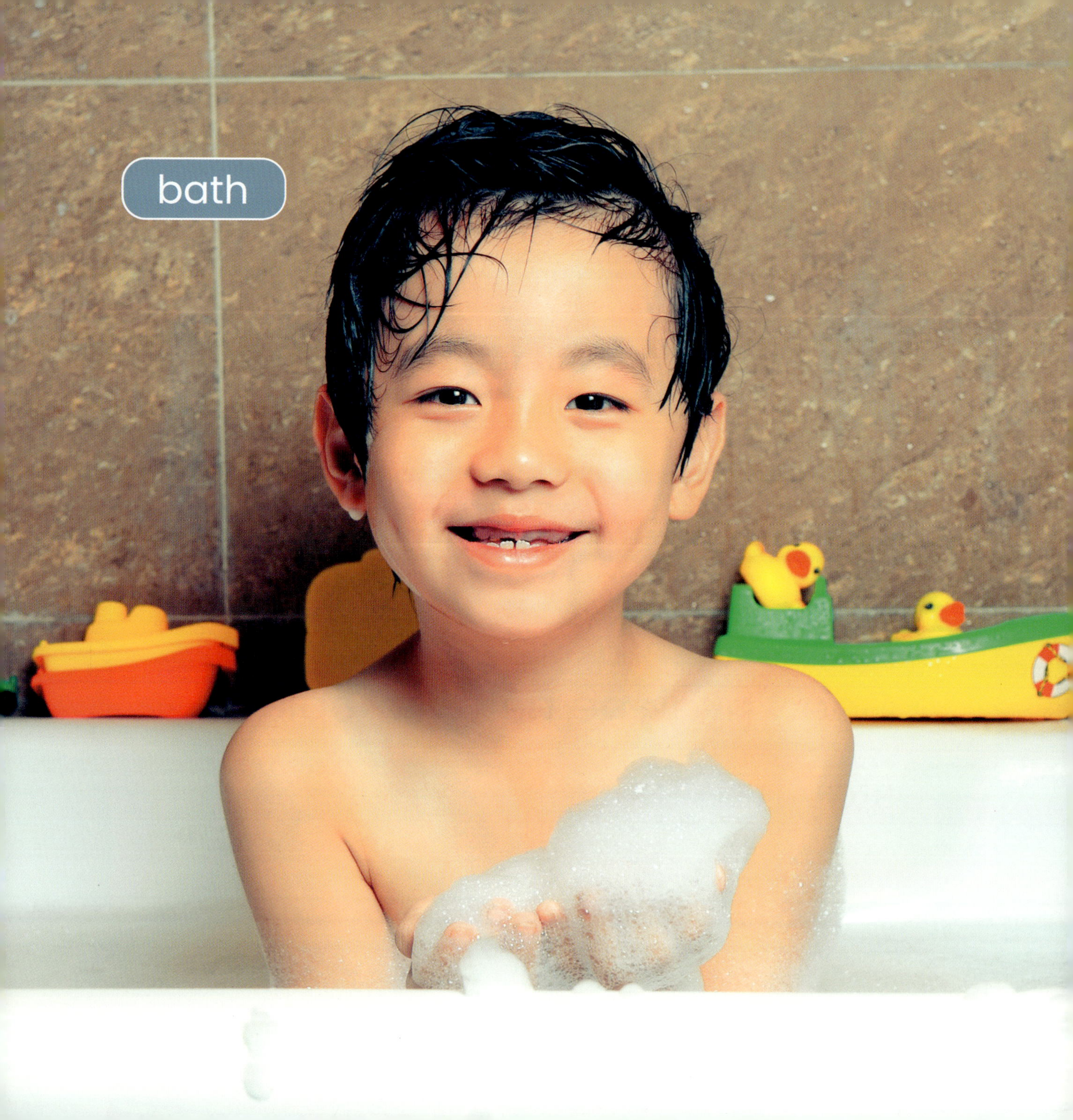
bath

Washing

Washing the body and hair is good hygiene.
Take showers or baths, and use warm water and soap.

Dry off with a clean towel. Then put on clean clothes. This includes clean underwear and socks.

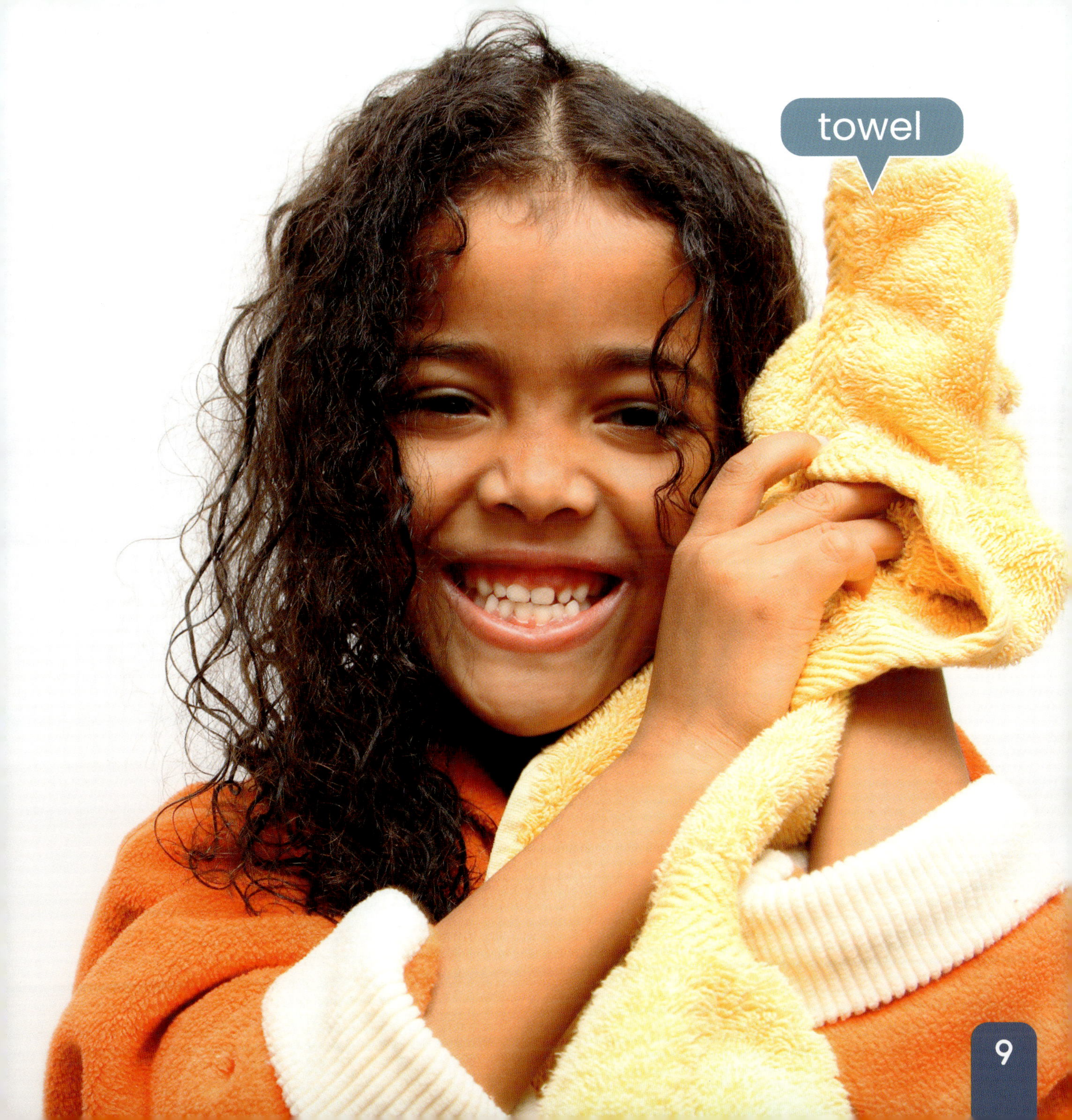
towel

Washing hands stops germs from spreading. You should wash after using the bathroom and before touching food. Wash after sneezing or coughing, too.

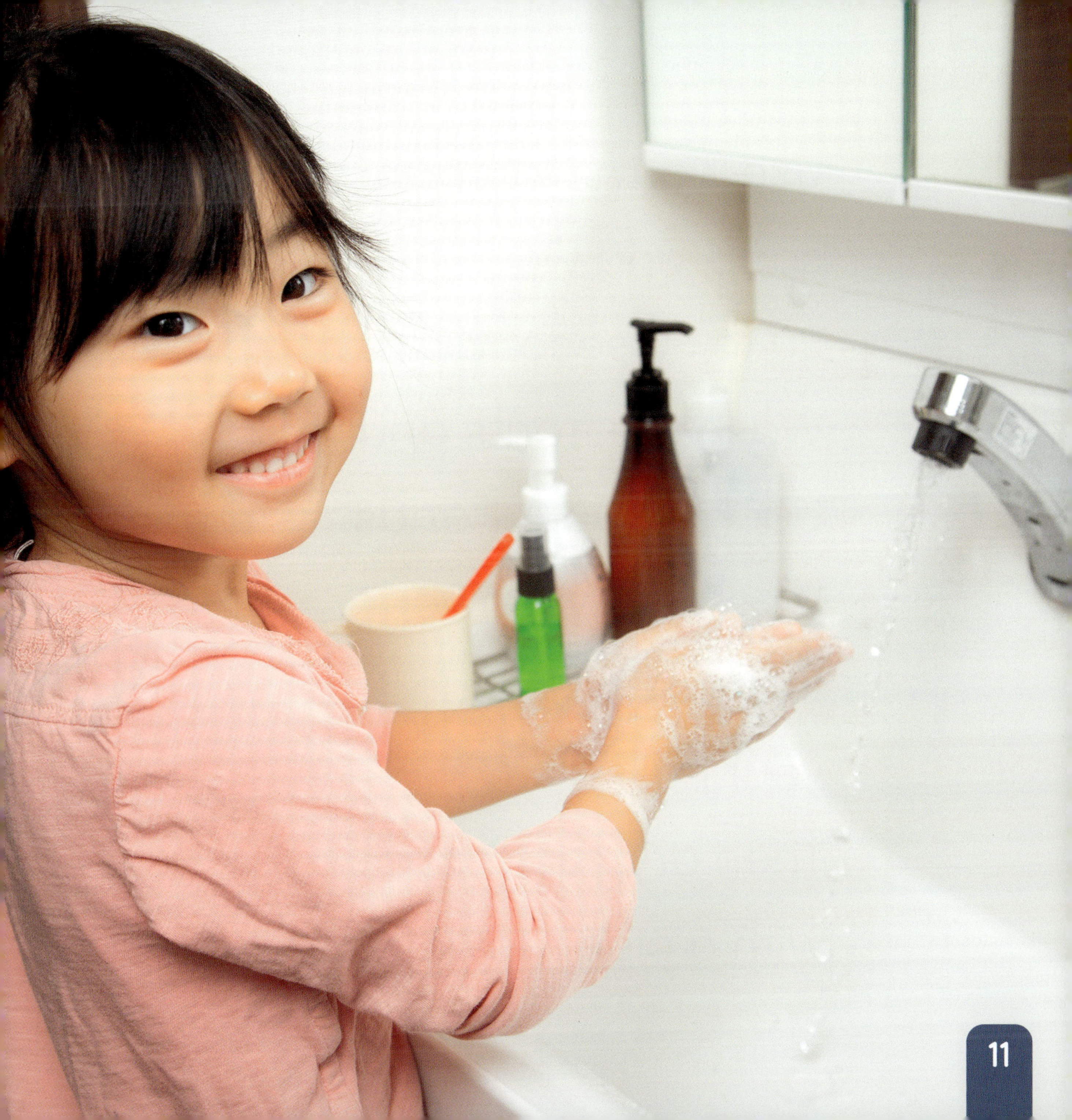

Use warm water and soap, and wash for 20 to 30 seconds. Wash the fronts and backs of your hands. Wash between your fingers and around your nails. Then dry your hands with a clean towel.

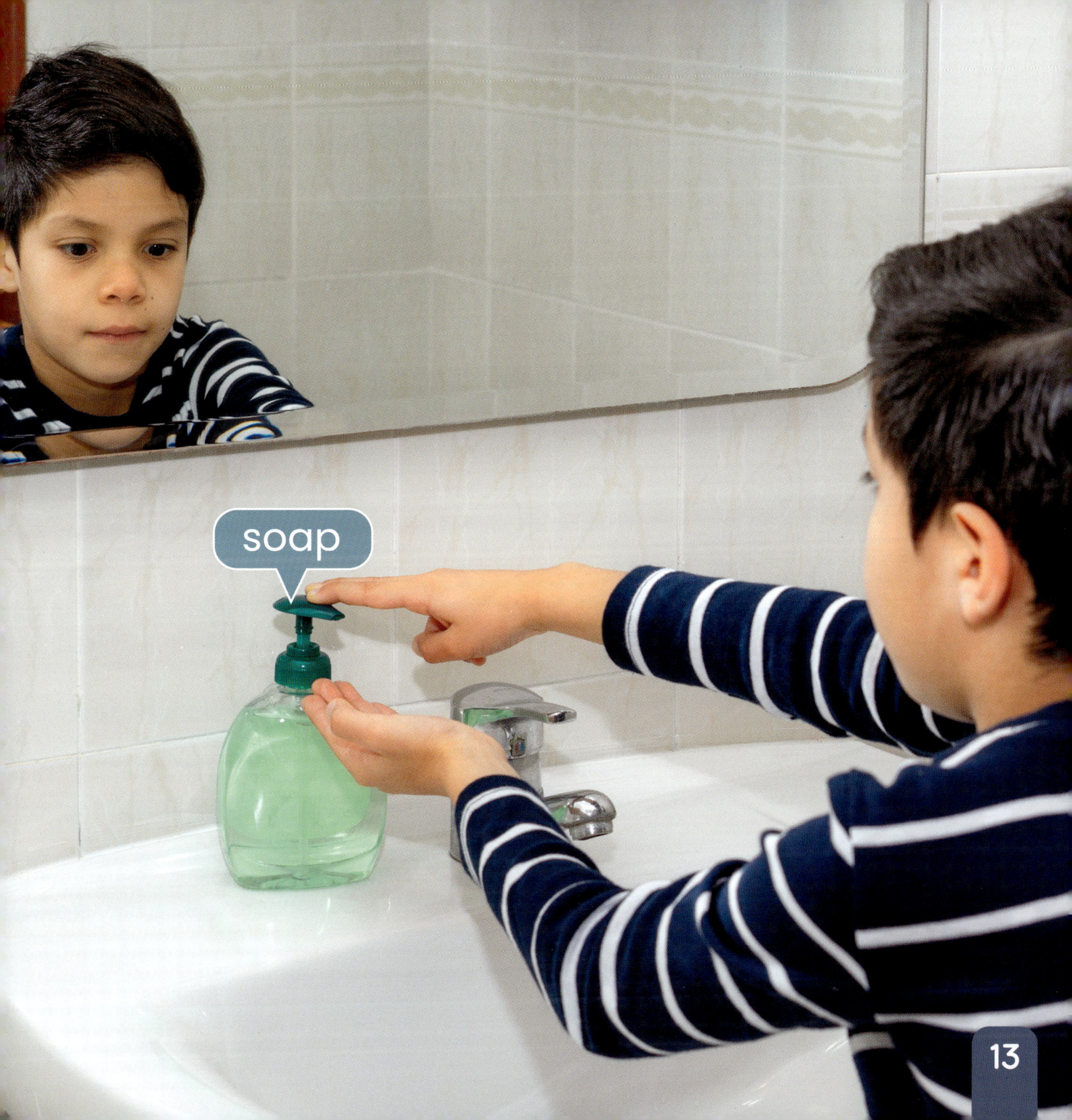
soap

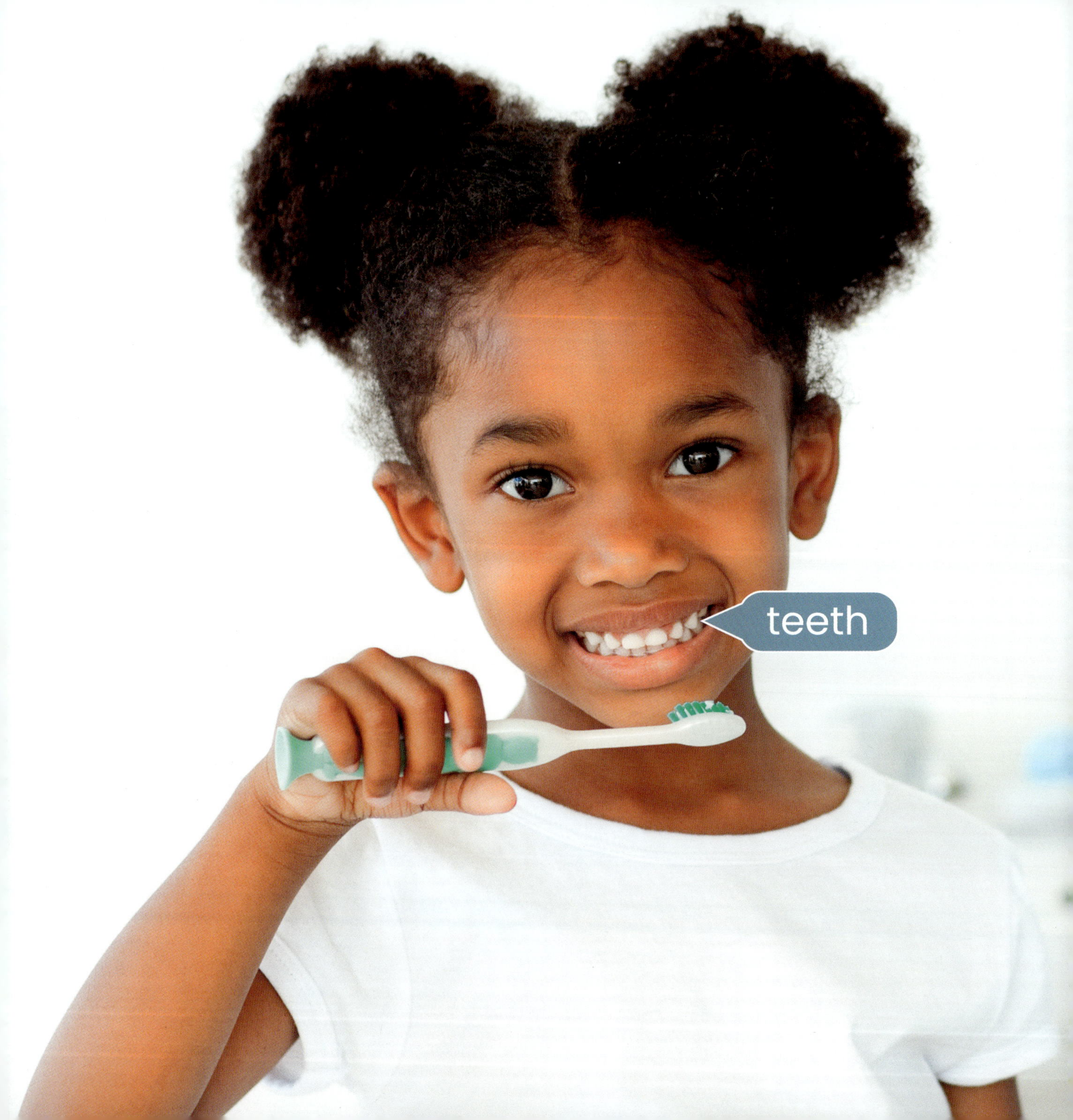
teeth

Brushing

Brushing your teeth is good hygiene. Our teeth help us chew food and speak clearly. They also give us nice smiles.

Germs can make teeth weak. Brushing keeps germs from sticking to teeth. It's good to brush at least twice a day. Brush after breakfast and before bedtime.

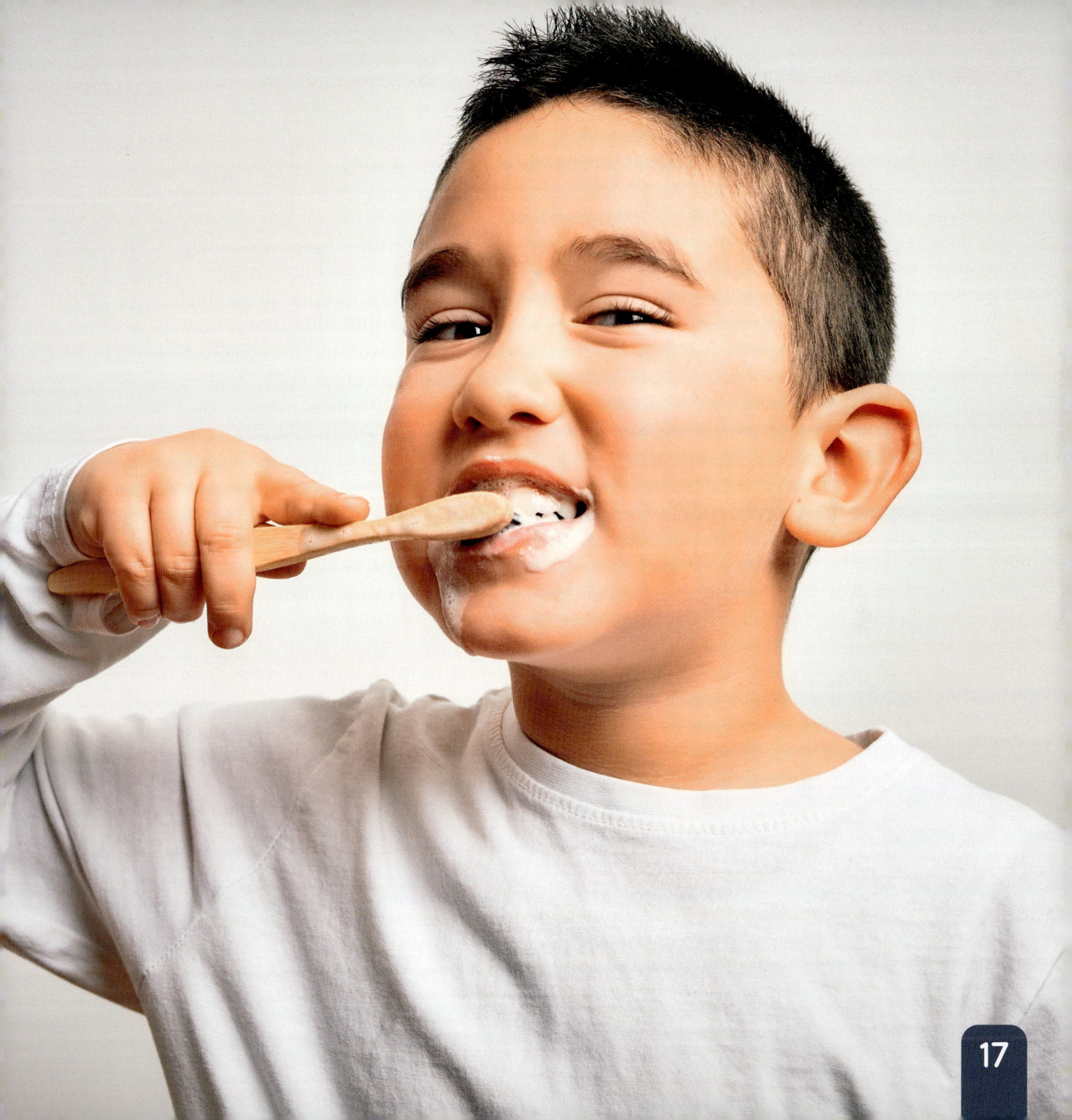

Put a small bit of toothpaste on a toothbrush. Brush for two to three minutes, and brush all sides of your teeth. Then spit out the toothpaste. A dentist can teach you the best way to brush.

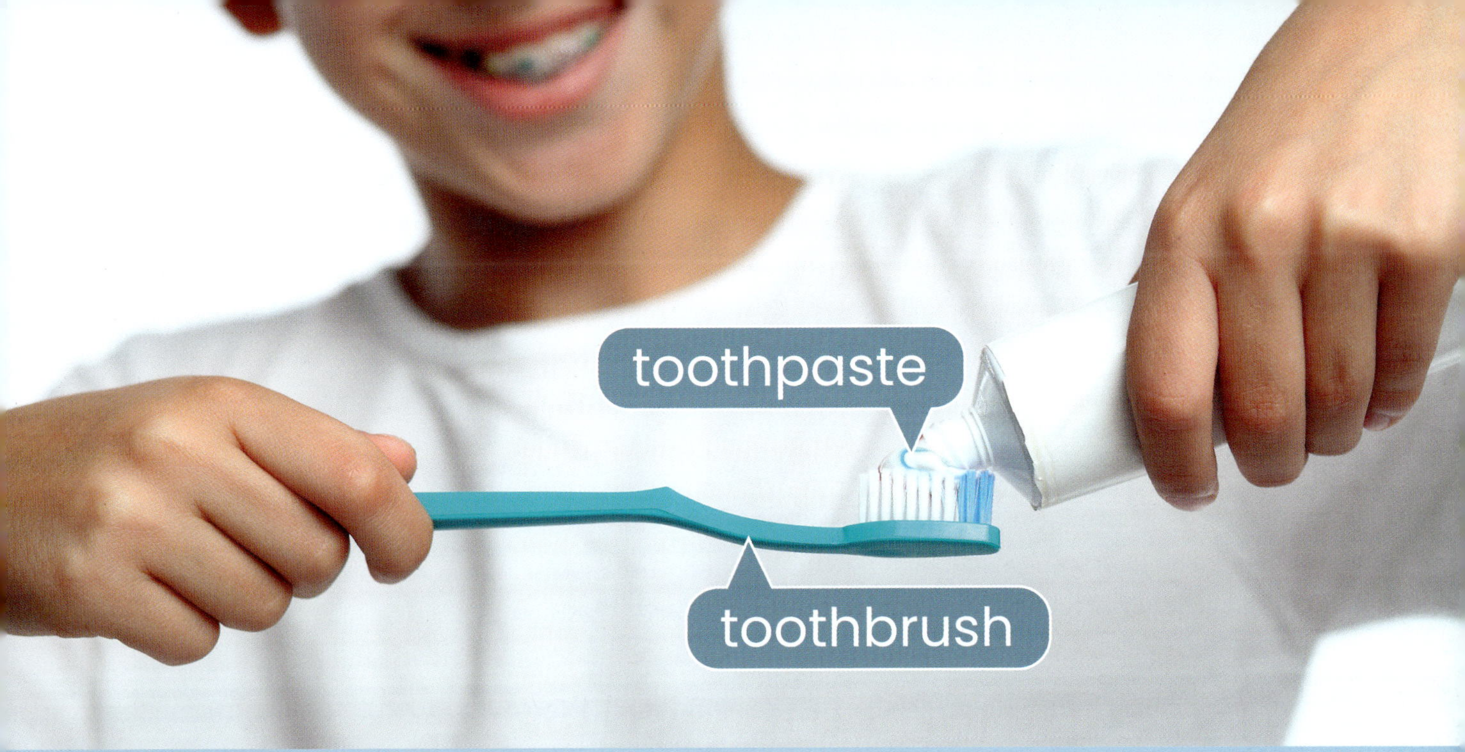
toothpaste
toothbrush

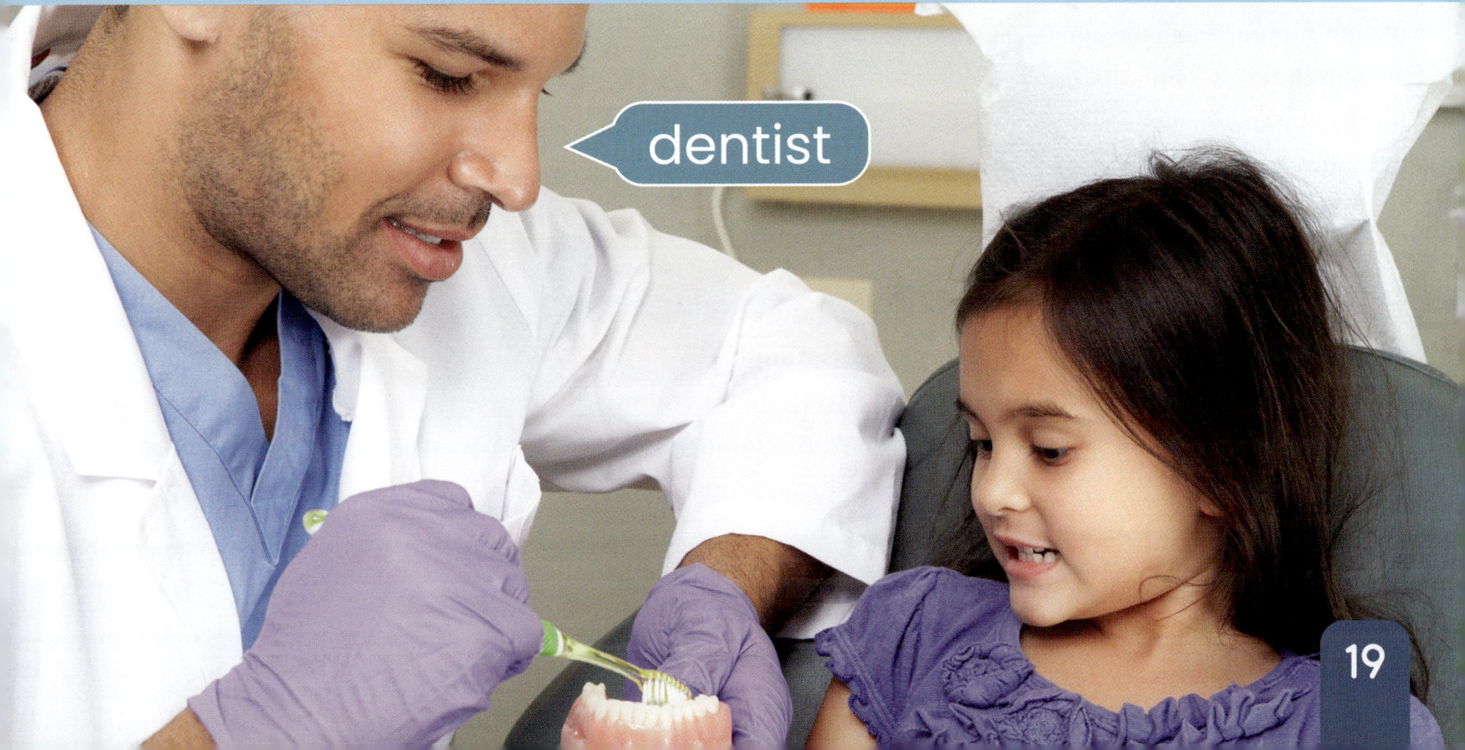
dentist

Flossing is good hygiene, too.
Flossing protects and strengthens the gums.
The gums hold the teeth in place.
Ask an adult for help with flossing.

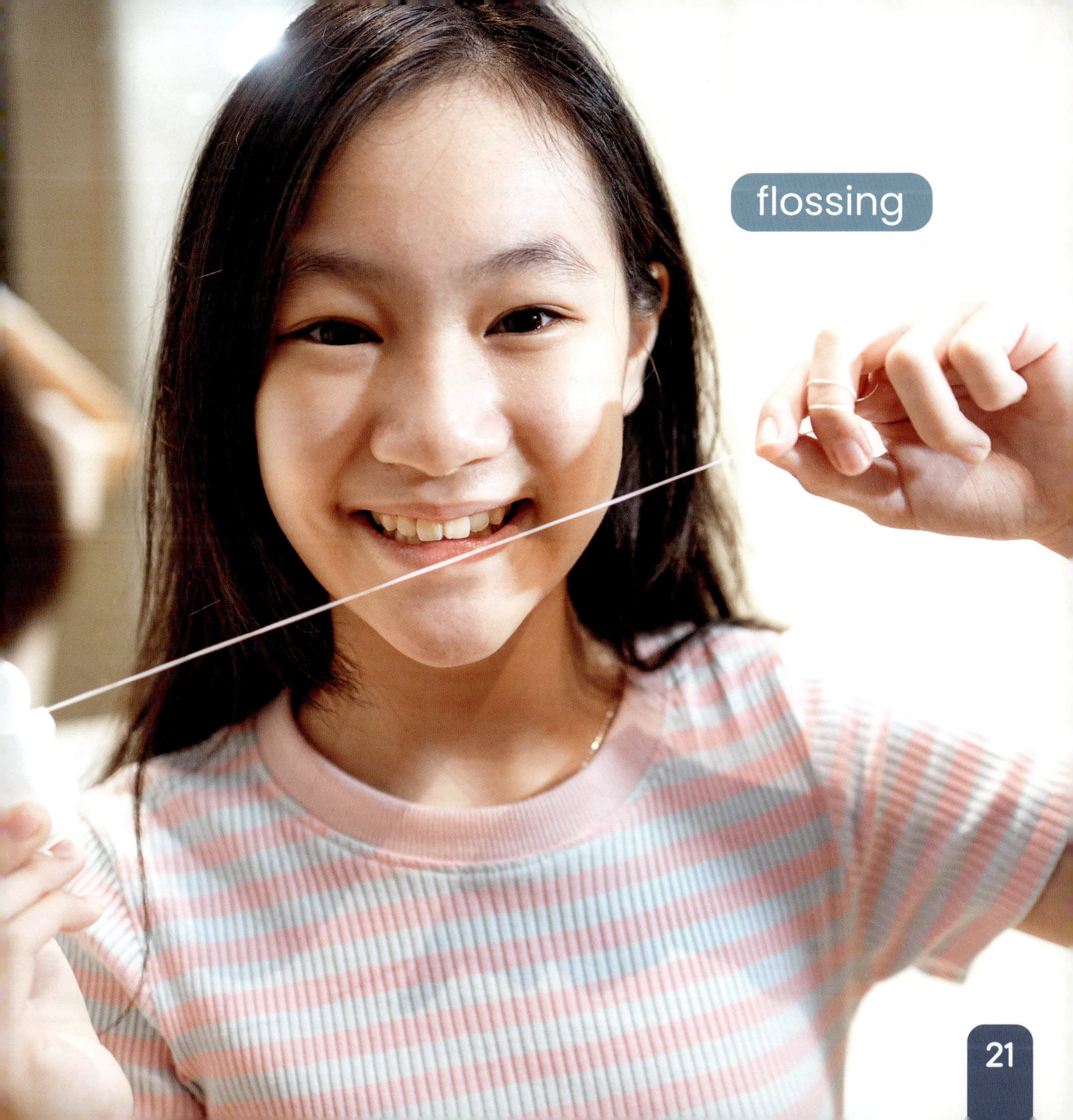
flossing

Washing, brushing, and flossing are all good hygiene. Practicing good hygiene will keep you clean and healthy.

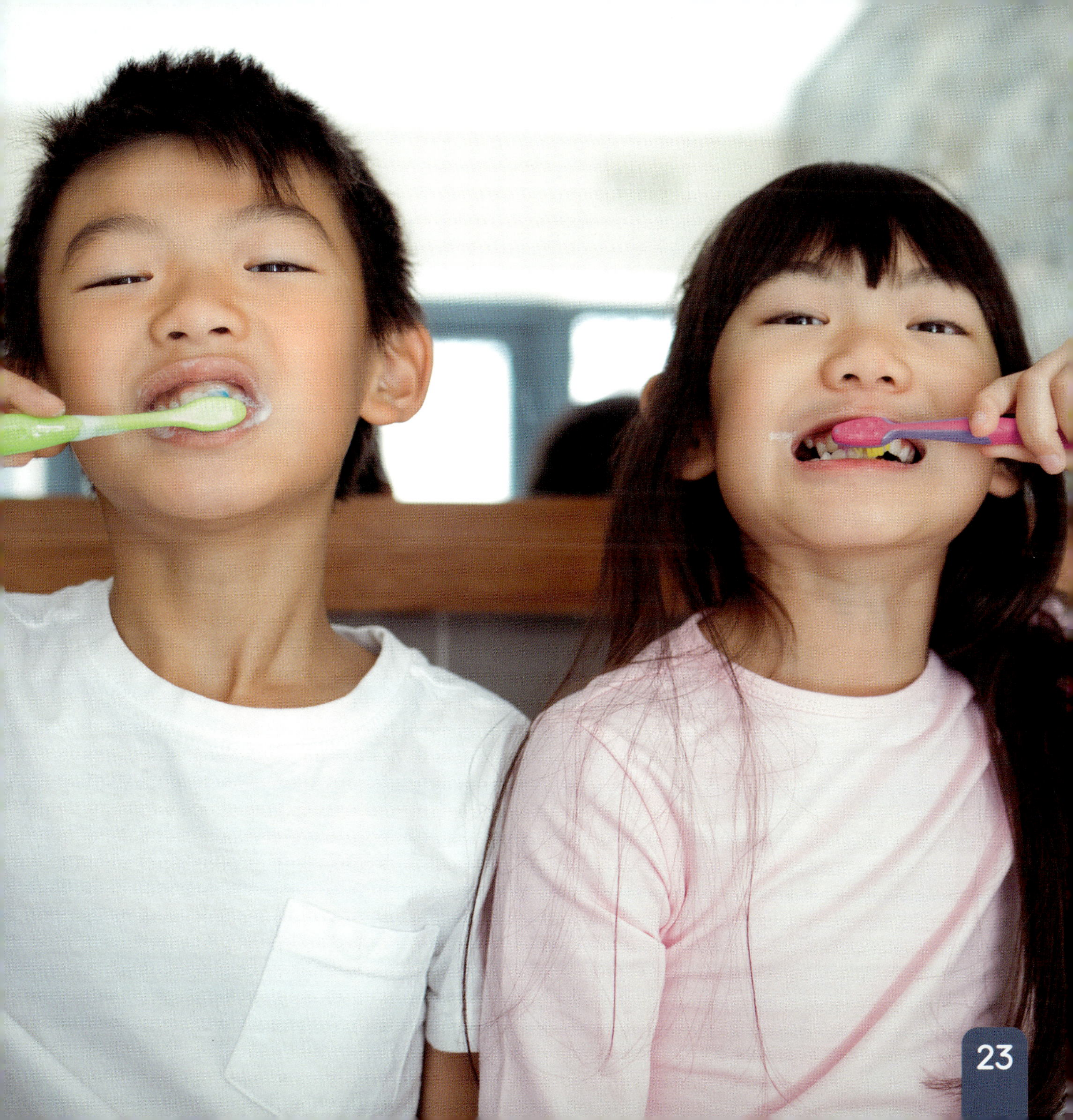

Glossary

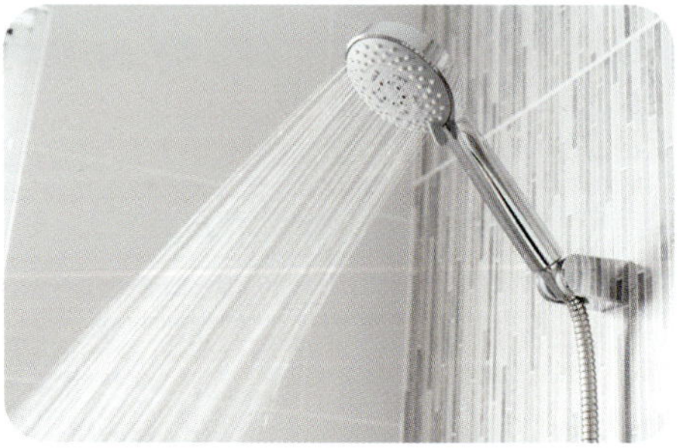

shower

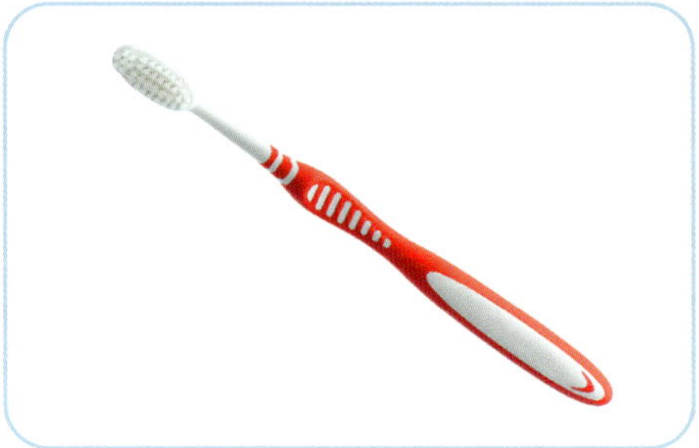

toothbrush

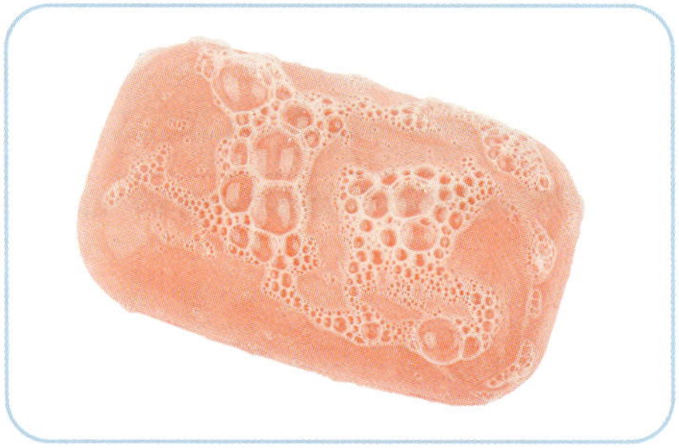

soap

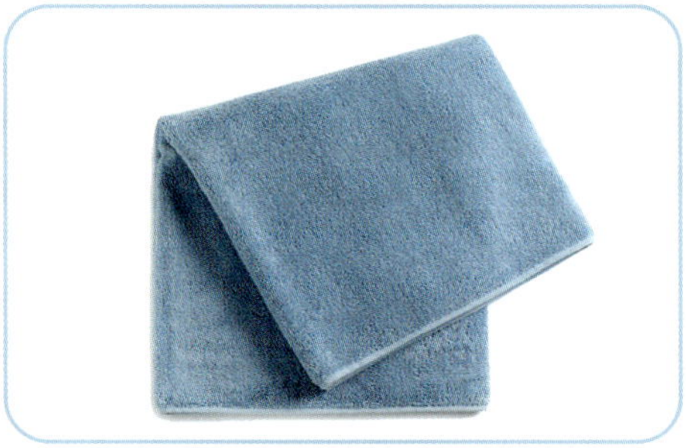

towel

Index